DEDICATION

This book is dedicated to my three adorable kids. Thank you for always taking care of your mother when I am not around

TABLE OF CONTENTS

Do It Yourself Home Gym

How to be a Fitness Genius in No Time

By: Christian Miller

9781635013214

PUBLISHERS NOTES

Disclaimer – Speedy Publishing LLC

This publication is intended to provide helpful and informative material. It is not intended to diagnose, treat, cure, or prevent any health problem or condition, nor is intended to replace the advice of a physician. No action should be taken solely on the contents of this book. Always consult your physician or qualified health-care professional on any matters regarding your health and before adopting any suggestions in this book or drawing inferences from it.

The author and publisher specifically disclaim all responsibility for any liability, loss or risk, personal or otherwise, which is incurred as a consequence, directly or indirectly, from the use or application of any contents of this book.

Any and all product names referenced within this book are the trademarks of their respective owners. None of these owners have sponsored, authorized, endorsed, or approved this book.

Always read all information provided by the manufacturers' product labels before using their products. The author and publisher are not responsible for claims made by manufacturers.

This book was originally printed before 2014. This is an adapted reprint by Speedy Publishing LLC with newly updated content designed to help readers with much more accurate and timely information and data.

Speedy Publishing LLC

40 E Main Street, Newark, Delaware, 19711

Contact Us: 1-888-248-4521

Website: http://www.speedypublishing.co

REPRINTED Paperback Edition: ISBN: 9781635013214

Manufactured in the United States of America

CHAPTER 1- INTRODUCTION ON D.I.Y. HOME GYM

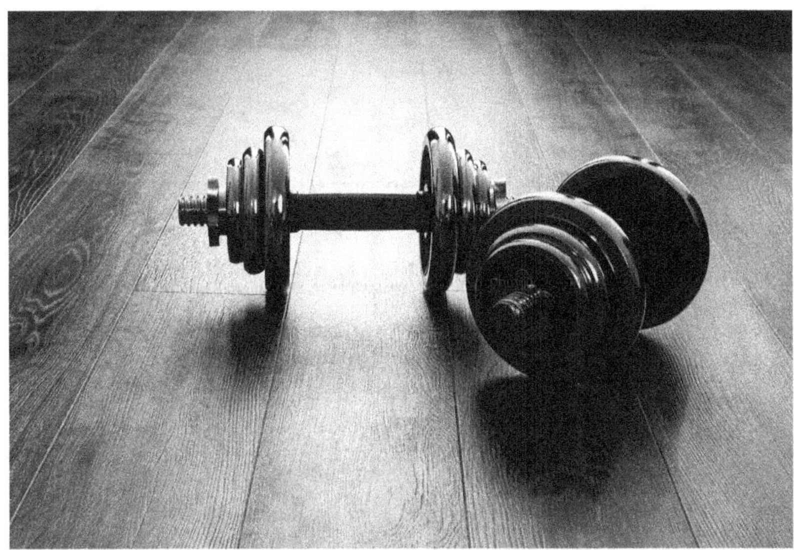

Today, more and more people are becoming conscious of their figure. But because they're so busy running their lives and their businesses, they don't have the time for workouts. Although local gym membership is very accessible and provides all the needed equipment for workouts, still conflict arises. It can include adjusting to the gym's opening times, stress of traveling from your home to the gym, and pressure on the weather condition.

In case you are facing this difficulty, consider building your own home gym to achieve your fitness goals and keep you in shape. There are various ranges of exercise equipment you can utilize at home. Time and weather conditions are not a problem anymore. You can do your exercise within your own set schedule. But the question is what equipment are you going to buy?

If you are starting out your venture, or becoming active again after a long break, it is advisable not to pursue your home gym. Instead you must enroll at a local gym within a short period of time. It can help you check out a number of fitness equipment available in the market today. You can ask your fitness instructor about its advantages and disadvantages and how the equipment can meet your fitness needs. Thus, you can list down the equipment that you will purchase for your home gym.

If weight training is your main focus, then the first step is to purchase a set of weights. You can buy free weights which are less expensive. The prices can be as low as $50 or lower. But you need a combination of weights weighing 4.5 kg (10lb) and 9kg (20lb) which is a hand-held dumbbell with a bar. The end of this bar is replaceable with other weights for more flexibility. There are different types of bars. But it is up to you to choose whether you are going to use the plastic or metal weights. Metal weights are the traditional weights used even before but plastic weights are more modern and often are sand-filled weights.

You can consider weight machines if you want to work out specific groups of muscles including the biceps, deltoids, and quadriceps in a safer way. Moreover, free weights cannot provide good workouts for the hamstrings and calves muscle groups. However, you need to pay the price of a weight machine. Costs and configurations may widely vary from a simple resistance machine, to an adjustable, multi-stationed weight stack. You can spend hundreds or thousands of dollars.

A stair stepper is another popular alternative. A simple stair stepper model can offer you a better cardiovascular workout and low impacts on your joints when exercising to build your calves and thighs. This machine is also a space saver and can cost from $80 to $150. A more complex stair stepper has adjustable speed, resistance level, speed, pedal distances and more. It also includes an HRM (heart rate monitor) as well as digital readouts for distance climbed, calories burnt, and speed. It can cost $1,700 to

$2,000. Treadmills are good workouts machines too for your home gym. The prices depend on the types, models, brand, and features.

Building your home gym will cost you money. However, it is worth investing to meet your fitness needs.

Choosing the Right Home Equipment

Today, increasing numbers of people are not getting more and more concerned about their physical health. Because of the increasing numbers of cases of heart related diseases, diabetes, and obesity, you have the right to be concerned about your physical well-being. This is why many people are now enrolling in gyms and are now starting working out as part of their daily routines to get and maintain a healthy body and healthy heart.

Besides, through exercising, you will not only have a healthy body and healthy heart, you will also obtain a great looking body that you can be proud off. In fact, many people exercise in order to have a better looking body. You can never deny the fact that a good looking and muscular body produces more sex appeal and is considered to be more attractive than having that extra flab or too thin. Having a great looking body also produces indirect benefits to you, such as having more self-confidence and a significant increase in self-esteem.

Health benefits and physical appearance are the two main reasons why more and more people are considering working out. However, what if you find working out in the gym boring or embarrassing. Many people get insecure about working out in public and for this reason they simply don't continue their workout routines at a gym.

Remember, you can still workout even if you don't go to the gym. The machines you see at the gym can be obtained at a very affordable price. There are home fitness equipment that you can purchase and use right in the comfort of your own home. Home fitness equipment can work wonders for you and get that great looking body that you have always wanted of having. Most home fitness equipment available today is designed to be compact to suit small homes, even an apartment. It can be folded and stored neatly when not in use and it can provide that same high quality workout that you would get in a gym.

If you are a full time parent where you always need to keep a constant lookout on your kids, you can consider getting home fitness equipment where you can both take care of your body and watch your kids. You will also enjoy your workouts because you can watch your favorite TV shows while you work out.

These are some of the home fitness equipment available in the market today. With the right home fitness equipment, you will be able to get a high quality workout and get that healthy and great looking body you have always wanted.

Factors When Shopping for Equipment

There are a hundred lots of home fitness equipment nowadays that are sold in the market. Do not make the mistake in buying something and then regretting why you bought it after a day or two. Home fitness equipment varies and you should always have one good reason to buy it. Don't believe everything commercials tell you about the equipment. Some equipment may seem easy to use on television but in fact will not really work for you. Try to ask yourself first of these questions before you grab your wallet and buy that equipment.

1. Do you need it?

The equipment should suit your interests and needs. The activities that you will do with that equipment should be challenging and something to enjoy on. Buying equipment is never a guarantee that you will use it especially if it is something new that makes it harder to use. Make sure that you already know the equipment and that it is something that you already tried in a fitness club. Start from buying small equipment that is aligned to your interests.

2. Can you afford it?

Don't be fooled with the thought that you will be forced to use something because you spent too much money for it. Expensive equipment is never an assurance that you will use them or that they are effective for you. Always consider how much you are willing to pay for certain equipment. Also ask yourself if it is worth it. Always check on the quality before you buy equipment. The price may be too low but consider that the quality can also be low. Or it may be expensive but then the quality is not that good. You can try choosing on cheaper alternatives but not sacrificing the quality of the equipment.

You may also want to check out for some used equipment. Most of the time, this is where you find a better deal. You can even find equipment that does not seem to have been used at all. Or you can find the equipment 3 months old but the price is almost half the original.

3. Do you have enough space for it?

This is often what buyers forget to consider. Before you buy something, make sure you know where you will place it. Your place may not accommodate the equipment. Plan ahead and make sure that the equipment can be placed in your home without causing any hassle.

4. Is it safe for you?

If you have existing conditions, be sure to check with your doctor to make sure that the equipment will be safe for you. Some equipment may be painful to use and might cause harm to your body. So make sure to try it first before you buy it.

It also suggested that you first consider if a gym near you already has that equipment. You can save money by just registering to that gym and use that equipment compared the price you will spend if you will buy that product.

Buying fitness equipment should be bought with consideration. Do not buy by impulse. Always ask the opinion of a professional gym instructor before you buy something.

Chapter 2- Fitness Equipment for Your Body Needs

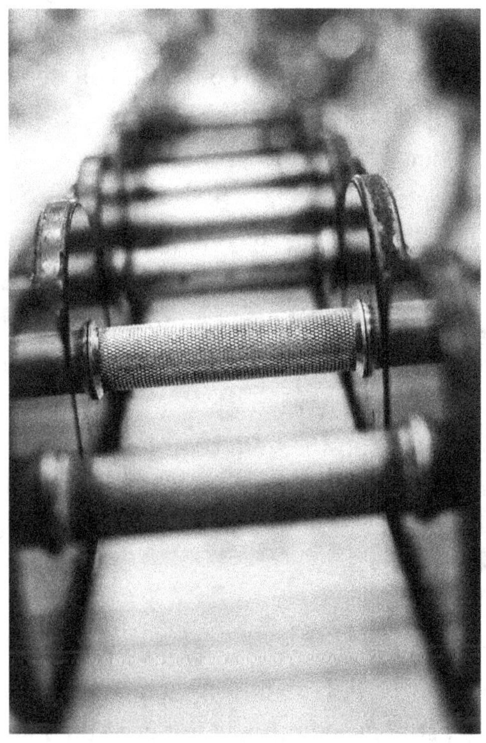

Today, more and more people want to have a great looking body for different reasons. Some people wants to have a great looking body in order to attract the opposite sex, some wants to have a great looking body for health reasons, while others simply enjoy working out.

There are several methods that people use to get a great looking body. You have to consider that not all of these methods are considered healthy. There are people who are too lazy to exercise and try different weight loss methods ¢with negative results to their bodies; some try liposuction surgery. You have to consider that lIposuction is only a temporary method. You still need to maintain your body by exercising in order to prevent it from accumulating fat again. You have to realize the fact that muscles burn fat. The more you exercise and develop your muscles, the fatter you burn.

There are also people who try different diet methods. People come to the point where they don't eat anything at all and this method can have negative results in your body as it can deprive your body the nutrients it needs. The best way to lose weight is by eating right and combining it with the proper exercises. With the hectic lifestyle that people have today; they often neglect their body's health because of work. The next best thing you can do is by purchasing home fitness equipment. There are different kinds of home fitness equipment available in the market today and different kinds of manufacturers. Because of this, you have a wide variety of fitness equipment to choose from. You also have to realize that because of the different home fitness equipment popping out of the market today, people tends to get confused on what to buy and often end up purchasing fitness equipment that they don't even need.

In order to buy the right fitness equipment, you need to know about the different types of fitness equipment available in the market today. First of all, you should not base on brands alone. The first thing you need to do is be familiar with the different fitness equipment available.

Cardiovascular exercises are one of the most important exercises. This is why your first fitness equipment purchase should be for the cardiovascular exercises, such as treadmills, cross-trainers, and elliptical trainers. When the time comes that you need to develop your muscles, strength training fitness equipment, such as weights, are responsible for developing specific muscles in your body.

Of course, it is natural that you have to have fitness equipment that will last a long time. So, purchase a cardiovascular and weight training fitness equipment with a brand that most people use and have positive user reviews.

These are some things you need to consider when purchasing fitness equipment. By knowing about the different fitness equipment, you will never go wrong with any fitness equipment you buy.

Smart Tips for Equipment Shopping

How do you regularly stay fit, healthy and flexible? A hearty diet of nutritious fruits and vegetables is the key as well as regular and continuous exercise. The best exercise is one that you are really and sincerely going to be working out on, be it push-ups, stretches, jumping jacks or the regular jogging or the much tamer walking. However, there are people who prefer to work out using fitness equipment in their own homes.

The following are a few basic and important things to consider when buying those exercise equipment.

1. Do not believe what you see and hear

At least not everything, it is good if you assess all those claims exercise equipment declare in their advertisements. It is so hard to accept as true for example some statements that assure people that they will lose several pounds off their weight in as little as seven days or that you will decrease your pants size in one month. Even with the assistance of dietary supplements, it is not possible to accomplish changes as major as these in just a few weeks, much less days.

2. Fat Burner is a No Burner

Be skeptical about claims that say you will be able to burn a tremendous amount of fat in a specific area of your body, such as the hips, thighs, waist just by applying a specific type of ointment or lotion, etc. The only sure way to burn all those fat way is by changing what you eat. Exercise is the best solution to works out every area of the body whose fat you want to get rid of.

3. The only testimonial that counts is yours

Before and after pictures of people who claim that they were able to lose weight because of using such and such equipment, may or may not be true. If ever they are, their experience is purely personal and that is no assurance that your unique body weight, body make-up will also undergo the same change they went through.

4. Read the fine print

It is always advisable to read the fine print of anything. Though you believe that the fitness equipment you are planning to purchase is a good one, reading the fine print really wouldn't hurt as it may say that you also have to decrease your calorie intake and not just rely on what the machine could do for you.

5. Do the math

There are advertising statements that say you could pay off the fitness equipment in a number of easy payments or by paying a mere $39.95 a month. Do not forget to inquire about shipping and handling costs and include that in your calculation. Also, add-on the required sales tax, delivery fees, set-up fees. Know all the details before you purchase.

6. Guarantee the warranty

It is best that you consider asking about details on their thirty day money back guarantee. Though this could sound good to you as the consumer, it may or may not actually do you good if, for example, you are going to return the item. You may actually pay for the humongous shipping cost and it could cost you more than what you could guarantee to receive in thirty days.

7. Call customer service

Make sure you contact their customer service hotline. Usually, they have toll-free numbers that you must be able to easily contact as well as a customer service representative who must be glad to be able to take your call and answer thoroughly all or any questions you may have about their products and services.

Building Muscle: Free Weights vs. Bulky Machines

Strength training is excellent for developing different muscle groups, and there are plenty of machines that will aid you in your fitness regimen. You need to make comparisons between using exercise machines and free weights. Both have its advantages and disadvantages and the purpose of comparing is to weigh which one meets your fitness needs the best.

The latest construction of free weights is widely available in the form of barbells and dumbbells. Many dumbbells are single weight, one piece items. Some are designed similarly with barbells. It has a bar in the center and the weights are removable. Thus, it gives you the option to change weights. This is less expensive, however time consuming. You need to replace weights for every exercise.

Weigh stack machine have two types, single exercise (created for one movement) and multiple exercise machines (adjustable for performing various exercises).

Free weights are beneficial for strengthening the entire body. Oftentimes this is more effective. Exercises on free weights are done easily; you properly hold the free weights while standing. Your entire body is supporting the weight that is why the muscles actively move during the exercise. This also supports bone mineralization, significant in avoiding osteoporosis in the future. As you lift the free weights, weight stabilization also takes place keeping your body in a steady manner. This promotes additional muscle strength.

The major advantage of training machines over free weights is safety and easy usage. These machines are equipped with control and guides to direct the resistance paths. Thus it is less dangerous and prevents the user from being pinched, injured, or trapped. In case you failed to control the weights, the stacks will never hit you. The spotter's assistance is not anymore needed when exercising. Heavier weights are more comfortable to lift, increasing your muscle mass. Adjustments on the machines can be easily made that is why this machine is very popular in many fitness centers and gyms.

The free weights major disadvantage is safety. If you perform a bench press using a barbell, the tendency of being trapped is possible especially if you fail to complete a certain repetition. It is advisable to do your exercise with a spotter or a friend to assist you. Keep in mind that greater amounts of control are needed when stabilizing your muscles. Total control is needed when lifting to prevent joints and muscle injuries.

Usage and technique must be properly applied when utilizing free weights.

Many manufacturers have created resistance machines with different qualities and designs. Most often these machines are for typical users with typical heights, limb lengths, and weights. The motions of the exercises are guided by these machines. So, sometimes the motion cannot be the perfect motion for the limb length and size of your body. This forces your body to adapt such motions which are not actually good, making your exercise useless.

The choice depends on you. To summarize, free weights can be better for achieving full stabilization of the muscles and freedom of motions, while machines provide safety and easy usage. Consider your fitness goals and choose accordingly.

Work the Body, Not the Pocket

Today, more and more people are getting more and more concerned about how their body looks. You can never deny the fact that having a great looking and muscular body is very attractive. With those well- defined muscles, you can be sure that you will have more sex appeal than your average person with that extra "love handles" or "beer belly".

Having a great looking and muscular body means that you will also have a healthy heart. First of all, you need to consider that muscles burn fat inside your body. By doing this, you will be able to prevent heart related diseases where fat clogs up your arteries and makes you suffer from heart attacks and strokes.

You have to realize the fact that there is a significant increase of heart related diseases and diabetes cases in the United States. Thanks to fast food and automation, people in the US are getting fatter and lazier each day. More and more Americans are turning their TV off, and are now starting to exercise in the gym.

Exercising is the best and the normal way to develop your muscles and keep your heart healthy. It is very important to remember that by exercising, you will be able to have that muscular body you have always wanted. What if you don't even have time to go to the gym and you prefer staying at home?

You can consider answering this question by purchasing your own home fitness equipment. You also need to realize that home fitness machines are quite expensive. If you are a type of person who is at a lower income level and you still want to exercise, you can still do so by jogging around your local park.

The main disadvantage of this is your local weather. If it rains or snows, you can never go out and do your daily run. The best way to exercise without going to the gym is by purchasing used fitness equipment. Some people sell their equipment because they plan on replacing them with newer models, while other says that they sell their equipment because no one actually uses it.

However, before you purchase used fitness equipment, you have to consider the fact that the equipment is already used and may have maintenance problems. If it is possible, you have to try it out first for a few times.

By doing this, you will determine if the used fitness equipment being offered is still in good working condition. Never buy used fitness equipment that emits strange and unnecessary noise when being operated.

If at all possible, you can bring your fitness trainer along when shopping for used fitness equipment. They will be able to determine if the used fitness equipment being offered is in top working condition or not.

They will also be able to recommend some fitness equipment that you need.

Chapter 3- The Ups and Downs of the Fitness Ball

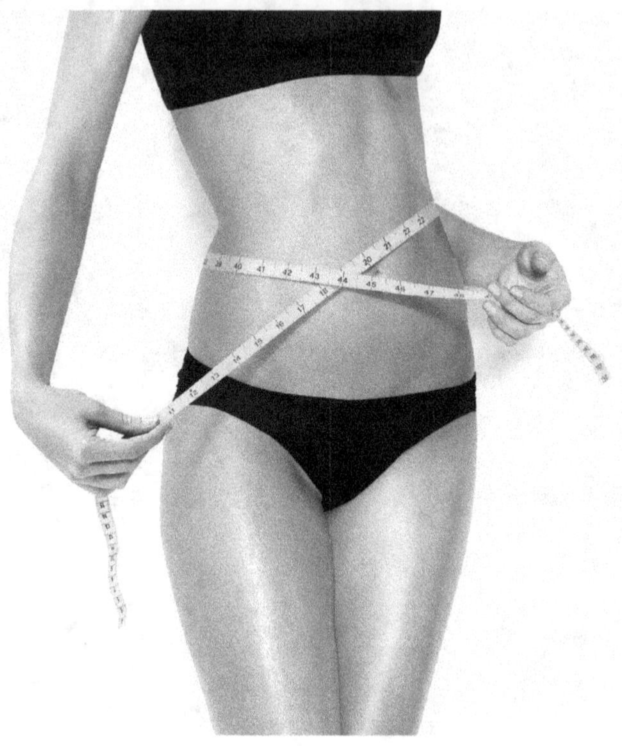

Most people dream of getting into shape, losing weight, and exercising more. It can mean signing up at local gyms. However, many fitness enthusiasts prefer to purchase home fitness equipment that can be effective for them.

They can take the benefits of a total workout while at homes and within flexible times. One of the best options to consider is buying a fitness ball. It is the time for you to experience a unique workout at home. There are various reasons why this equipment has become very popular. In fact, it is utilized by most physical therapists to treat their patients from back pains.

A fitness ball having a diameter of about 55 to 85 centimeter is made of elastic rubber. It is utilized in exercise and physical therapy. There are various names for a fitness ball such as exercise ball, Pilate's ball, gym ball, therapy ball, balance ball, body ball, yoga ball, sports ball, and Swiss ball.

The major benefit of a fitness ball exercise is enabling the body to respond to the ball's instability while keeping the balance and engaging the muscles as well. Keep in mind that the muscles are strengthened upon struggling to maintain the balance. The core muscles of the body, back muscles, and abdominal muscles are the target of the fitness ball program of exercises.

Exercises done on a fitness ball will never bore you. In fact it can challenge your stamina, patience, perseverance and self-discipline. This is the true form of exercising, working the entire core muscles to achieve the best results.

A fitness ball is effective because of its rounded shape. It can create instability to induce your core body muscles to work. Compared to floor crunching, the muscles that are only working are the upper abs, but when you do the crunching on a fitness ball, the core muscles including abs muscles, back muscles, pelvic muscles, and hip muscles are working together in helping you stay on the ball.

Try doing a few push-ups using fitness ball, your hands on the floor and your feet on the fitness ball or vice versa. This exercise gives more stability when the feet are spread apart and tougher when the feet are put closely together.

Although a fitness ball provides many advantages, there are also some pitfalls especially if overused. Strength coaches revealed that it can cause injury and approximately 70 percent of fitness ball exercises are considered worthless. Nevertheless, it is still prescribed by some therapists in treating patients with back pain.

Incorporating a fitness ball in your fitness program can mean surpassing all the difficult levels involved during the exercise. Each requires support from your stomach muscles and back to help in keeping the trunk muscles firm. More often, a fitness ball is good for people who have lower back pain. Other uses include developing overall strength and control of the body's core muscles, increasing the strength of back and abdominal muscles, learning proper posture and body mechanics when lifting objects, and increasing mobility of the lower back.

Suit Up for an Active Life

The world is getting more and more competitive every day. In order to keep up with such competition, every individual should focus on their body's fitness. For some, it can be a simple walking or running exercises while for others, it may mean months spent in fitness gyms.

There are different kinds of fitness activity. Some activities require certain equipment, but there are also activities that don't require any; but there's more to just fitness equipment. A great number of people are more concerned with the right fitness apparel that will suit their exercise activities. This is the very first step to achieving fitness. In today's times, sportswear and fitness apparel flood almost all stores that sell such items. You can find bras, shorts, to full fitness outfits. Most people are able to conduct their fitness exercises effectively if they look great. In choosing your fitness apparel, there are certain tips to follow when buying such outfits.

Motivation is needed in order to be truly committed if you want to achieve all your fitness goals. There is a need to choose the right fitness apparel that will work for you in doing your fitness activity. Looking great has its advantages and even if other people don't understand the correlation between fitness exercise and fitness apparel, this is a fact that you're bound to follow to achieve your goals.

Since there are many forms of workout, you have to choose the most common activity that you're consistent with. For example, you're into aerobic exercises. You can find a lot of suits that go along with this type of exercise. You can buy it from any local department store or apparel store; or you can also check online stores if they offer such apparel. If you love doing yoga, you can also choose from a wide selection of tank tops and pants.

Experiment on color combinations so that you can get the most out of your several existing clothes. Individuals who happen to be spinners can get some shorts, matching halter, and bra or tank top. Women just love to dress up, and this is not only true to special occasions. Even if you're going out for a fitness activity, it really helps a lot to look and feel good about yourself. These garments are one of the important keys to achieving a physically fit body although not necessary.

As you go through your fitness regime, you can easily notice any changes in your body if you wear the right fitting clothes. By seeing instant results, you will be more motivated to pursue such activity. By wearing form-fitting clothes it can help you in checking whether your body's in great shape or not.

When you go shopping for your fitness apparel, it is best to find flexible clothing that can aid you in carrying out all your physical activities efficiently. Don't practice carelessness by ignoring fitness accessories like fitness apparel. But as an educated buyer, you don't have to fall victim to attractive advertisements. They only offer expensive clothes when you can always find a good buy if you only do some research and window shopping. Quality and price are two very important factors to consider when purchasing your fitness apparel.

Active Wear

In a sports apparel specialty store you will delight at the wide range of clothing plus accessories that is available in the market. Specific sporting apparels like golf, fitness exercise, equestrian and yoga are very much available. The apparel for sports like surfing or rafting and even mountaineering are abounds. The wetsuits are perfect for surfing apparel. The sports apparel includes caps, batting gloves and rafting vests.

Here's a short list on how to choose your sports and fitness apparel

1. The Golf wear

The golf apparel can be found in any specialty sport store. The golf apparel usually includes a trouser with a t-shirt. In golf, comfort is the most important factor. Chinos are also very popular golf wear. Hats and caps of varying designs and makes are also available. Of course outlandish gears worn by some professional golfers are also available.

2. The Running / Fitness wear

Running apparel is best made with cotton to retain moisture that causes friction and might lead to possible chafing. The shorts and tights including the cotton socks are basic running gear. When running apparel is being chosen, try to select a base layer top which keeps you dry for an extended run. Comfortable and fit running shoes must be matched to keep you fresh on the run. The fitness gear pertains to all kinds of apparel including aerobics and gymnastics. The multi-colored tights and leotards are the best and most comfortable during a workout. The fitness gear must be selected with care. The proper material and correct size is a must when selecting the fitness gear.

3. The athletic apparel

The athletic apparel must be chosen with the climate and weather in mind. An apparel that is not suited for the weather will hinder the performance of an athlete. A popular athletic wear is the running or jogging pant with a drawstring waist. These types of athletic apparel can be purchased at discounted rates. The all weather gear is designed to keep most of the elements out. An athlete depends on the athletic gear to perform at his best.

4. The Equestrian apparel

Equestrian gear is mainly about breeches and boots. There are specialty equestrian stores that stock clothing and other equipment for riding. The casual equestrian gear could be riding breeches matched with a plain shirt. The paddock boots available also at equestrian apparel stores complete the set for an equestrian. A pair of riding pants and a jersey can be bought at an equestrian apparel store. When having lessons on riding, you may want to look online for equestrian stores to see and choose an outfit which lets you ride with great style and comfort. A little pricey in most cases but may be worth the price. A western style of gear is also available in specialty shops.

5. The Yoga apparel

Yoga apparel must be very comfortable and loose for easy movement. A t -shirt and a loose-fit short are basic yoga apparel which will keep you fresh and comfortable. Also, it does not cost much. Designer yoga apparel is also available at special yoga stores. Yoga Capri pants and unitards are available at yoga apparel store. The special Asana clothing can be found at very exclusive yoga outlets!

Choosing the Right Fitness Club

Fitness clubs are effective motivators. They should motivate us and not frustrate us. Before you choose a fitness club, make sure that it suits your needs and goals. You should first learn and decide on what are your priorities, then, you will know what you need in a fitness club. Here are some guidelines you can consider in choosing a fitness club that is best for you:

5. Where is it located?

Location is the first thing that you should consider when finding a fitness club. If the club is far from your home, you'll use it as an excuse not to work out. It is best to find a facility that is near your home.

6. Are the employees friendly, nice and willing to help you reach your goals?

Make sure that the instructor has the necessary experience to work with you. The instructor should be a certified professional that can work with you safely and effectively. Your instructor should also know if you have physical limitations or you may find an instructor that is well trained to work with you. You can also check the age of the instructor especially if it is one factor for your motivation and learning. The staff should also be helpful, friendly and professional. You can also ask the services they offer and find what is important for you. Some facilities have their own dietician and physical therapists that can offer services for you.

7. What kind of programs does it offer?

Find time to see what programs are there for you and check if they suit your interests. Do they offer group classes? Choose the facility that offers the classes you really like. You can do a trial class to check it out if you want.

8. Are the facilities and equipment good and will they be available anytime that is most convenient for you?

Check if the equipment is enough for all members. Otherwise, you will waste your time falling in line and waiting for your turn. Also make sure that the facility is open during the time you are most likely to do work outs and exercises.

9. Is the entire facility well maintained, clean and safe for you?

Machines and other training facilities should be in clean and good working order. If you see a lot of "out of order" signs, it could be something to think about. Modern equipment is safer and more comfortable to use, so you may also want to consider that. Are the floors cleaned regularly to avoid accidents? Is there enough room for everyone?

10. Are the members of the club friendly and can they become your friends?

The fitness club is also a venue for social interaction. Take time to drop by and meet the members of the club before you enroll. Other members can be your buddies in the near future and should be considered.

11. What is the schedule of classes and will they be convenient for you?

Find out what classes are offered at a specific time and consider if you will be available at the schedules given.

12. How much would it cost you?

It is important to know the monthly membership fee and what it covers. Some fitness clubs have hidden charges and you should be keen in checking that. Check if they have promotions or discounts and do they offer services at an extra fee. It is also important to know how long the club has been and how often they increase rates.

13. How is it different from other fitness clubs?

Don't just stick to one fitness club. Try to visit as many facilities as you can and make a comparison. Then you can narrow down your choices to the facilities that met your needs and priorities.

14. What do people say about it?

Take your time to gather feedback from other members. Ask them what they can say about the club and let them tell you about the experiences with the facility.

Choosing a fitness club is just like shopping on the best shirt for you. Do not be pressured and do not try to contact them right away. You can take your time to review and gather enough information if you are still not sure which one to choose. Once you have made your choice, enjoy and make the most out of it.

Chapter 4- Your Fitness Club is a Reflection of You

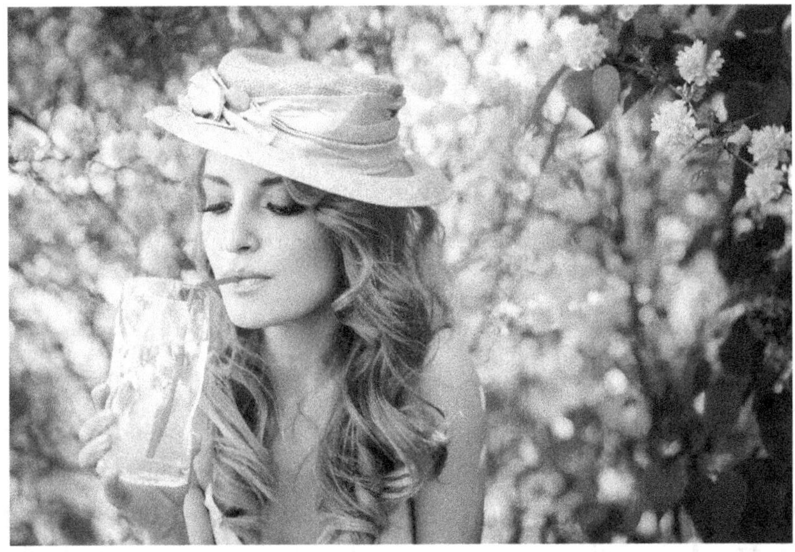

In reality, you really do not have to spend a lot of money on expensive health club or fitness center memberships, treadmills, or the latest fitness gadget to get moving. However, some people find that if they make a monetary investment, they are more likely to follow through on fitness.

Fitness centers are, basically, built to provide people the proper fitness equipment, trainings, and other devices needed to keep an individual physically fit.

However, not all fitness centers are created equal. In fact, there are fitness centers that require their members to sign some contracts, which in the end will not be easy to cancel. Hence, it is important to know the characteristics of the fitness center that will work best for you.

Here is a list of some tips that you can use:

1. Make your mind up on things that you need

Before you choose a fitness center, you should first know what your needs are as far as physical fitness is concerned. This will determine the kind of fitness center that you will find. For example, if you are into sports fitness rather than the typical physical fitness activities like aerobics, then it would be better to choose a fitness center that has sports facilities and not just treadmills.

2. Do not forget to shop around

It may sound like a cliché but it really pays a lot to a person who shops around before deciding on something. Hence, when choosing fitness centers, it is best to do some shopping first and get to compare the prices, charges, and the facilities available in a health club. This way, you get to choose the best and yet affordable fitness center you could ever find.

3. Consider your budget

It does not necessarily mean that just because you have plenty of money, you will eventually give in to a fitness center that you have first encountered. It is best that you have a budget to follow so that you will know where to focus your finances before you decide on signing-up for a fitness center. Just remember, you want to work out for your body and not working out something that you will soon be in debt just because you forgot to stick to your budget.

4. Know where your money goes

If it makes you sweat and lose the fat, fine! Make sure that whatever fitness center you have chosen, it is important that you get what you have paid for.

5. Be wary of the physical attributes and characteristics of the center that you wish to enroll in.

Make sure that the fitness center that you have chosen is clean, properly ventilated, and complete with all the amenities that you need. Be sure also that the equipment the fitness center has are all in good working condition. Never use fitness equipment that appears to be worn out. This will only cause more harm than good. All of these things are boiled down to the fact that a fitness center does not have to be a perfect fitness center. What matters most is that the fitness center that you have chosen is good enough to generate good results in your body.

The Fitness Center is Your Playground

Maintaining a physically fit body is vital to being healthy. Fitness centers can help us to keep in shape. In a fitness center, you would find lots of equipment in which you can physically exercise.

Below is a listing of the equipment and programs commonly found in a fitness studio:

Treadmill

This is a piece of sporting equipment that allows the user to run without actually moving a distance. The word treadmill is used to refer to a kind of mill which is run to grind grain. The treadmill operates by the principle called belt system in which the top side of the belt runs to the rear so that the runner could run the same distance. Therefore, the speed of the treadmill can be measured or set since the rate of the belt equals the rate of the runner.

Weight training

Weight training is under the strength training program designed to develop the size of skeletal muscles and physical strength. It uses the principle of gravity; the trainee's force would be used to oppose the pull of the earth. This weight training makes use of different kinds of equipment to develop specific groups of muscles. Dumbbells, weighted bars or weight stacks are the most commonly used.

Cycling

Cycling is commonly done by people who want to improve their cardiovascular health and fitness. In this view, cycling is particularly beneficial for those suffering from arthritis and for those who are not fitted to play rigid sports like running which require strength of the joints.

Swimming

Swimming is a very good exercise. Swimming is also usually recommended for those who with disabilities or who want to rehabilitate after injuries.

Racquetball

Racquetball is a sport game where racquets are used along with a hollow rubber ball. This can be played either in indoor or outdoor courts. Unlike other racquet sports like badminton and tennis, the usage of the floor, ceiling, and walls of the court is legal instead of out-of-bounds. Two players are involved in the game, although some variations of this game have three and four players.

Aerobics

Aerobic classes usually include stepping patterns, done with music and signals directed by an instructor. Research shows that aerobics is one of the healthiest exercises. Aerobics, literally meaning "with oxygen", helps the body to use and consume oxygen more efficiently by training the lungs and heart. This helps to reduce stress and to control weight.

Basketball

While this very common sport is an indoor game, other variations have been popular as this sport can also be played outdoors.

Yoga

Yoga focuses on meditation. It is considered as a way to both spiritual and physiological mastery.

Martial arts

Martial art is structures of arranged traditions and practices of combat training. Martial arts today are not just being learned for combat purposes, but also for fitness, self-defense, mental discipline, self-cultivation, and character development.

Physical therapy

Physical therapy deals in maximizing and identifying movement potential in promotion, treatment, prevention and rehabilitation. This includes services that are concerned with circumstances where function and movement are threatened by injury, disease, or ageing.

Fitness Center Membership Terms

When a person needs improvement, they think of a much better way to achieve their desired results. For example, get fit and maintain it by considering a health club membership. But doubting sometimes cannot be denied since a lot of stories can be heard regarding people who have already signed up. They are active for more than two sessions and never showed up again.

It is very complicated to purchase and maintain a membership in a health club. But there are guidelines that can help you save money and achieve your fitness needs.

1. Set up your priorities by listing specific fitness wants and needs.

It can include options such as joining a large health club that is open for both males and females, getting access to other clubs, joining an exclusive service for personal training, assessing the frequency of workouts every month, thinking of how to maintain a fitness regimen, and budgeting the money for paying a monthly health club membership.

2. Visit the health clubs once you requirements are identified.

Take advantage of the free passes from these clubs and workout more often upon free periods.

3. Never sign up a health club membership unless your free passes are over.

Sometimes managers and sales people can pressure you and encourage you to sign up to take advantage of the discounted price. Don't be in a hurry since discount pricing is offered by health clubs all the time.

4. If you decided to join, talk to the sales person regarding membership choices.

Never be afraid to sign up a long term health club membership contract. This contract is an installment loan and paid with higher interest rates. But if you think you cannot maintain such payments, never sign the contract. Instead collect all written information and go home. Review it during your leisure time.

5. Ask the sales person everything you want.

Never feel pressured or rushed. Don't forget that your signed contract supersedes any sales person promises. Although everything is written in the contract, these are not legally enforceable. Carefully read the terms and conditions before signing.

6. Make comparisons with every type of membership.

Your ultimate decision must answer your needs not basically for availing the short term discounts. It may appear like you are saving money. However, in the end it can cost you a lot.

7. Make sure that cancellation requirements on the health club membership are fully understood.

Cancellation of most health clubs with long term contracts are often impossible. Choosing a monthly contract can be a good solution.

8. Never consider automatic payments through credit cards.

It can be very difficult to stop the payments once you have decided to cancel your membership.

9. Always check all your paid accounts.

This is important in case disputes arise with the health club.

10. When you cancelling your membership, make sure that you obtain it in written form. Making the right choice depends on how good you are in assessing these guidelines to benefit from all the advantages of a health club membership.

24 Hour Fitness Center Perks

The 24 Hour fitness center is your one stop shop to everything about fitness and well-being. Imagine it as the Wal-Mart of the fitness industry. All of them have equipment which caters to weight training, cardio vascular equipment and a variety of fitness gear is also available. 24 Hour fitness centers all have locker rooms and – believe it or not – some even offer babysitting accommodations. Over all, the 24 Hour fitness center is a complete, clean and extremely well maintained facility that can cater to all your fitness wants, needs and preferences.

It is very easy to get started on your path to fitness. 24 Hour fitness centers have over three hundred clubs located in the whole nation and are open for twenty four hours. There is no long term contract to sign up in. You have the option to pay monthly, but you are offered a complete personal training package that suits your body type, body weight and built so you are ensured with a service that is truly personalized.

Which club do you belong in?

24 Hour fitness centers give you the option to choose the specific type of club that you desire. The active club involves a group exercise as well as free weights and cardio machines to work off that fat. The sport club also includes everything in the active club but with additions such as basketball, heated pools and whirlpool. The super-sport club also includes the amenities found those in the active club and the sport club but with more additions such as massage, a sauna as well as a steam room. The ultra-sport club is the works. It includes most of the amenities found in the active, sport and super sport club, plus a day spa, courts for racquetball as well as an executive locker room.

The Path to Performance

It all depends on what you want to achieve. In 24 Hour fitness centers, a uniquely specialized fitness program is available to anyone who simply wants to improve their performance in a specific sport or is seriously training for competition. The program is designed by athletes.

The Performance program includes a menu plan specifically customized for those intense workouts. A resistance training is also available as well as a full cardio workout. After your exercise, a metabolic rate test is conducted.

This program is designed for those who want to get started as soon as possible but have no clear and specific idea how. This is clearly the best option because all the information on nutrition, resistance training is learned through the program. This is the foundation one needs in order to have the results that will last your body a lifetime.

The Components of Fitness

A regular or an intense workout is just part and parcel of your path to health, fitness and well- being. There are other factors that should just as well play a part and which 24 Hour fitness centers teach you.

Food is one of them. A menu is provided to those who follow the performance path. This details what you should or should not eat, or at least eat less of, if not completely avoid. Cardio is also one, as this enhances your endurance to stress and exercise. Vitamins and supplements are a necessity unless you are sure that you are able to receive the proper amounts of iron, calcium, vitamin C, D or E in a day. Resistance training is a feather in your fitness cap and is a necessary tool for being healthy, wealthy and wise.

If you like staying fit, you have to consider going to the gym or health clubs in order to stay healthy and maintain a well-toned body. However, you have to realize the fact that not all health clubs and fitness centers offer great quality services that will provide you with positive results.

When joining a fitness center or a health club, you have to make sure that the fitness club you join isn't only after your money. It should provide great quality service that will enable you to see positive results in the quickest time possible.

One kind of fitness center and health club is 24 Hour Fitness. They have different fitness programs for different people that will enable their clients to get results as quick as possible. 24 Hour Fitness is one of the leading fitness centers in the world. They only hire professional fitness experts in order to assist you with your workout needs and they also hire qualified nutritionists that will advise you on what kind of food you should eat and what to avoid.

They have programs that have been proven to be effective and they also offer their membership at a very affordable cost. They have different fitness programs for different people and they even have membership for the whole family. Their fitness plans are proven to be very effective and they have professional fitness trainers that can assist you, your family and friends to have a better body and a better health.

If you have experienced fitness centers where there are incomplete equipment and existing equipment are obsolete, rusty or difficult to use because of maintenance problems, you have to consider becoming a member of 24 Hour Fitness. They offer state-of-the-art exercise equipment and complete amenities that are well-maintained. This means that you avoid the frustration of working out in unreliable exercise equipment or waiting for your turn at a machine.

24 Hour Fitness can be found almost on every continent and you won't have any difficulty locating one. They also offer different kinds of workouts that will suit your needs and one that you can easily adjust to. 24 Hour Fitness is also a participant of the Passport Program where you can work out in other fitness centers. All you need to do is show your 24 Hour Fitness Passport Program ID, pay the fee and you can work out like you are a member of that particular club that is also a member of the Passport Program.

The Passport Program can be very useful if you are traveling and you can't find 24 Hour Fitness in that area. This means that you can work out anywhere in the world. With over 3000 fitness clubs all over the world that are participants in the Passport Program, you can be sure that you can still workout even if there isn't a 24 Hour Fitness Club near the area you are traveling to.

Beyond the Diet with Healthy Diet Recipes
Working out at 24 Hour Fitness is fun, easy and can provide you with positive results in your body and also in your health.

Americans are said to be the most unfit people throughout the world. This notion is rooted from the fact that many of the American populace suffer from obesity because Americans are fond of their fast food restaurants.

Good exercise is known by everyone as being vital in maintaining good health. This is more ideal when taken along with a good nutritional plan. The populace of the United States is advised by their doctors to lose their weights. In this way, they will be able to evade the other threats on their health, like heart ailments and diabetes.

As a result, 24 Hour Fitness centers have started to prosper. It is in this place where the term fitness is branded. In the United States alone, several numbers of 24 Hour Fitness sports centers already exists. What makes 24 Hour Fitness sport popular is the fact that it gives more time to do exercise. It's even more convenient for those who do not have the time of day or who work odd hours. The centers of 24 Hour Fitness sports, as its name implies, operates 24 hours. Because these centers give more time for people to exercise, they become more and more fond of it. In fact, more and more of these centers are opening up in the United States now. Americans appear to be addicted to fitness. They want to be fit and healthy.

The 24-Hour Fitness sports centers offer a multitude of activities: swimming, racquetball, spa, tennis, weight training, bicycling. The fitness instructors at these centers plan the appropriate exercise as well as nutritional plans suited for each client's needs. When your doctor gives you a physical report, you can present it to your fitness instructor. Your physical report will guide your instructor to design the best fitness program along with a nutritional plan that fits your needs. No doubt, 24 Hour Fitness sport centers help people to achieve their want of a beautiful body, here it can be achieve in a healthy manner. No need to undergo into liposuction to trim those fats.

Exercise is enough to burn them all in good shape. In addition, 24 Hour Fitness sports centers are also a place where one can meet and mingle with different types of people; a great place for socializing. This is also one of the reasons why more people are exercising in these types of centers, and why they make it part of their routines.

Chapter 5- 24 Hours Fitness Center: Very Flexible Hours

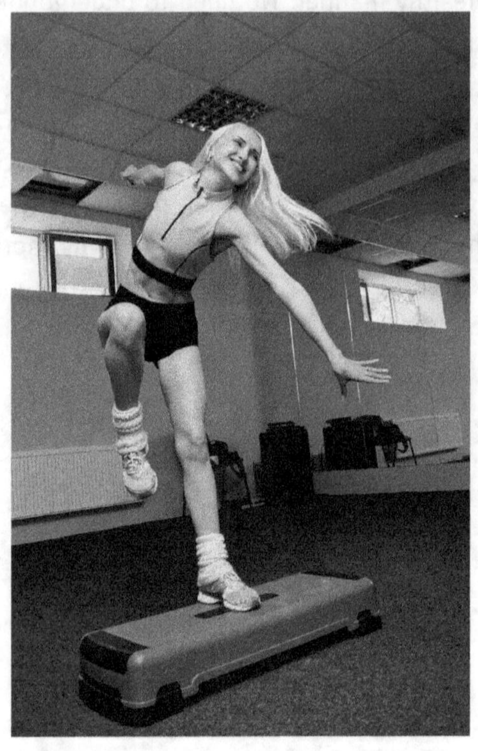

You can be sporty though you are not a bona fide sportsman and be healthy enough to fight disease; You can have fun and meet new friends, simply by having your exercise regimen at a 24 Hours Fitness center. 24 Hour Fitness centers offer all of these possibilities

This type of center presents flexibility; this has become the Mecca for many of its patrons. The fitness here, as its name implies, go for 24 hours. Here, the people who seem to be very occupied by their work still have time to ensure their health through exercise. Whenever they find time, they only need to go to the center and attend a class; even in the middle of the night, or perhaps, before dawn. The fitness class schedules are very convenient for the clients. According to the fitness instructors, the centers play a vital role in molding the attitude of its clients and should be given emphasis.

These centers also shape the strong willingness of its regulars and a developed significant moral conduct. They help in developing the self-confidence and determination of their regular clients.

However, these centers still prioritize on its significant contribution in building a physically fit body and good health to its clients.

The instructors believe that through shaping the moral conduct of their clients, it alone will provide enough motivation in to vigorously pursuing and achieving their goals. They perceive that the right amount of determination is more effective as compared to any of the finest fitness equipment available in improving the body. Just as the muscles become more firm, the amount of determination also gets more compact. And as the body achieves a beautiful shape, it is directly in proportion to the efforts that have been exerted during the training. Because of these facts, 24 Hours Fitness centers are undeniably popular now to more people. These centers play a big part in improving ones perception of their life. In a simple way, these centers develop the inner and outer strength of their clients. 24 Hours Fitness centers are high in quality when it comes to the equipment they use. At the same time, the fitness instructors always aim to meet the needs of their clients, especially for the amateurs.

Nowadays, a great number of people are greatly emphasizing the growing need of feeling good, looking good, and living longer. Scientific evidence has revealed that exercise and fitness are among the keys to achieve such ideals. If you're a person tagged as a 'couch potato' or if you have a deskbound job, you will need sheer determination, commitment, and dedication to incorporate exercise/fitness in your day-to-day routine. The truth is you're not too young, old, or unfit to start exercising. Regardless of gender, age, or your family role, you can expect a great deal from regular exercise

If you're not committed to it, you will get nowhere. Once you've committed to achieve the 24 hour fitness, you must start having a balanced diet combined with exercise. This will help in providing you generally with good health. Aside from that, chronic illnesses can be prevented as well as premature death or disability.

Some of the benefits that you'll obtain from practicing 24 hour fitness are:

- Improved health and well-being

- Improved appearance

- Increased stamina

- Enhanced social and emotional life

Oftentimes, physical activity isn't a part of an individual's daily life and so getting moving can be a big problem. Most of today's jobs require minimum physical exertion. Our society is mechanically mobile and machines do almost all the hard work. Many people prefer to observe how things are done for them, including children. Statistics reveal that more and more health problems like obesity, diabetes, and other health conditions are rising. But don't lose hope yet because preventive medicine still works. One very good preventive measure is to practice 24 hour fitness, so keep moving now.

If you want start your 24 hour fitness regimen, experts usually recommend getting a maximum of 30 minutes of physical activity. Make sure that you do it moderately every day. You can do cycling; brisk walking, swimming, and/or just keeping yourself busy with household chores and repair. If you think 30 minutes is way too long, then you can always shorten activities to ten minutes at a time as long as it totals to 30 minutes per day.

Following a program can be very hard for the average individual, so instead you must decide to change a huge part of your lifestyle especially your unhealthy ways. This way, you can incorporate permanently all the necessary factors that contribute to 24 hour fitness. As you use your muscles, you're actually contributing to fitness unknowingly. You can't achieve fitness overnight; you must be able to do it gradually. Move from one simple activity to a vigorous activity. However, if you have an illness like that of cardio, it would be best to check first with your doctor. The same is also recommended for people over 40 years of age with high risk factors. If you want to achieve 24 hour fitness that will last for a lifetime, you must have consistency. Enjoy your exercise activities and never think that it's an obligation on your part. Instead, think of it as a way to live longer.

FITNESS DEPOT: A ONE-STOP GYM

Having a fit and well-toned body also means having a healthy and sexy looking body. You have to consider the fact that because of the alarming increase of heart related diseases, obesity and diabetes, it is very important for many people today to integrate a health plan in their daily life by eating the right kinds of food and also by exercising.

Beyond the Diet with Healthy Diet Recipes

One of the most popular ways to get a healthy body and have your daily exercise routine is by exercising in the gym. However, there are also a lot of people who don't have enough time to go to the gym because of their hectic schedule. If you are a single or a full time parent, you have to consider that going to the gym also means that you have to leave your children at home or take them to the gym and not get the proper exercise because of minding your kids. Purchasing some home gym equipment where you can work out right in the comforts of your own home can ease some of these stresses.

There are different gym equipment retailers available all over the country and one of the most popular and also one of the most preferred fitness equipment retailers is Fitness Depot. They offer different kinds of fitness equipment of different brands. They have fitness equipment for cardiovascular exercises, strength training, and they also offer different accessories to make working out more fun and more enjoyable experience.

Fitness depot is the largest fitness equipment retailers in Canada and this company also offers gym equipment all over North America at a very affordable price. You have to consider that putting up your very own home gym will require you to invest a lot of money. Gym equipment is naturally expensive and you have to realize the fact that in order to have a proper full body workout, you have to purchase several pieces of equipment that concentrate on specific parts of your body.

Fitness Depot was founded by Marc Dubois and Edwin Cameron back in 1993. The first store was located at 40 Ronson Drive, Toronto, Canada. Because of the popularity, the company became North America's choice for fitness equipment and up until today, the original Fitness Depot retail store is still open.

If you want to build a perfect home gym that can give you a great looking body, you have to shop for fitness equipment with Fitness Depot. Here, you can be sure that you will get the perfect fitness equipment for you to build your very own personal home gym and get that body you want at a very affordable price.

Besides, the way you live your life will depend on your body's health. By investing in home gym equipment, you will also invest for a healthier and better looking body.

LA FITNESS AWARENESS

Many people have already realized the importance of employing physical fitness for the body, particularly those that have certain kinds of diseases, start exercising for the sole purpose of losing weight. When the pounds do not drop as quickly or as completely as they would like, they get discouraged and give up. If you take away any advice about exercise and certain illnesses, let it be this: Even if you do not lose weight, your investment in exercise is still paying off in reduced heart disease risk and better blood glucose control.

Moreover, exercise simply makes you feel better, both physically and mentally. Your energy level will rise and the endorphins released by your brain during exercise will boost your sense of well- being. The motivating factors here is that you should never give up before you really get started. You owe it to yourself to keep going.

With the start of the Internet, information regarding these fitness centers is gradually dominating the Internet. Take for example LA fitness. It has its web site readily available, 24-hours a day, to anyone who wish to get some information regarding physical fitness. LA fitness is a conglomeration of different fitness centers in the United States.

Since its inception in 1984, LA fitness, as the sole owner of the different fitness clubs in the U.S., has continuously operated and managed the different sports clubs in Arizona, Georgia, Florida, California, Pennsylvania, New York, Texas, Connecticut, Washington, and New Jersey.

It continues to grow and expand its territory as it plans to have 135 additional fitness centers and sports clubs in the country. It aimed to operate new techniques and services for their new markets. Therefore, for people who wish to know why LA fitness always rings a bell, here are some of the reasons why it became as popular as it is today:

1. Commitment to service

The best thing about LA fitness is that its management and staff are committed to bring forth the kind of service that their clients deserve. They provide their clients with facilities that are totally way above the rest. They also modify and develop their existing fitness equipment in order to give their clients the needed satisfaction as far as physical fitness is concerned.

2. Fitness programs

Another best thing about LA fitness is that they continue to provide their customers with the right and appropriate fitness programs that would truly drive their clients to a healthier life. They have incorporated the concepts of yoga, indoor cycling, aqua aerobics, Pilates, and kickboxing among others. They have also employed the utilization of sports activities as part of their health and fitness programs.

With their sports fitness, they also have their own tournaments and leagues, which foster camaraderie and sportsmanship among their members. In turn, these additional activities provide better alternatives to those who do not wish to be constrained on aerobic activities alone.

3. Revolutionary approach in aerobics

Like any fitness centers, LA fitness has its aerobic programs as the main attraction on their programs. The only difference that LA fitness makes is that they focus on utilizing revolutionary approach to their aerobics programs. This, in turn, provides their clients with a better way of losing weight and maintaining a healthy, physically fit lifestyle.

Best of all LA fitness provides optimum customer satisfaction to their clients from the very start that they enter their clubs and centers. Indeed, staying healthy and maintaining a physically fit body is possible in LA fitness clubs.

CHAPTER 6- LA FITNESS LIFESTYLE

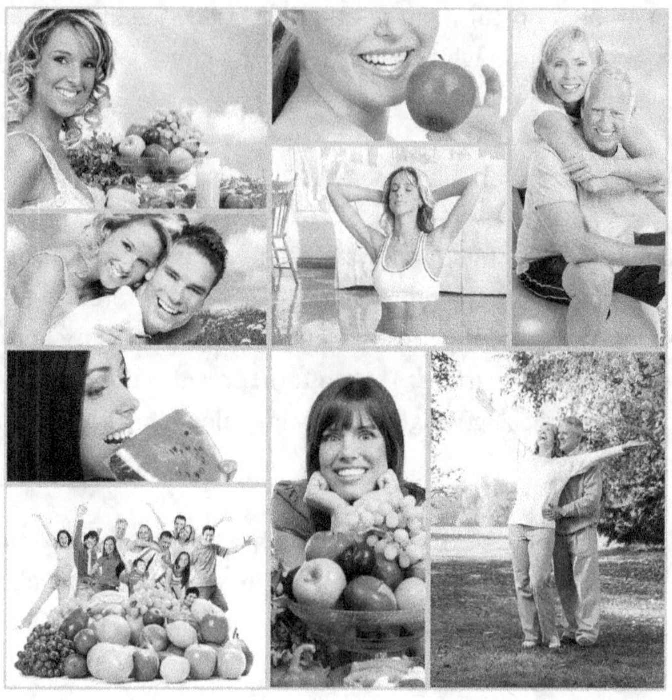

When you visit your doctor, they will always advice you to exercise and eat right. You hear this phrase almost every day from doctors, and even in TV and radio advertising. You have to consider taking this advice because it is very good advice. Exercising is the most natural way of losing that extra flab in your body and it is also the best way to keep your heart healthy. By combining exercise with the right kind of diet, you can be sure that you will be able to keep fit and healthy.

You can never deny the fact that exercising can be quite boring. You also have to consider the fact that exercising will not produce immediate and visible results after a few weeks of doing the same exercise routine every day. Because of this, people tend to simply give up exercising and just lie down on their comfortable recliner and watch TV all day. Besides, this is a better way to spend your day than getting tired doing exercise routines that doesn't even show any results, right?

If you answered yes then you are wrong. You have to consider that because of the alarming increase of heart related diseases, you have to consider starting exercising in order to keep your heart healthy. Exercising is needed by your body in order to let it function properly and not acquire any unwanted diseases. So, how can you make working out fun?

The answer to this question is by getting fit with LA Fitness. LA Fitness is a well-known fitness establishment that will provide you with all your fitness needs. They have fitness professionals who will be able to assist you with your workout. The best thing about LA Fitness is that they provide different kinds of fitness activities that you will surely enjoy.

If you enjoy swimming, LA Fitness provides pools for you to swim in. They also have racquetball courts and even basketball courts. You have to consider the fact that exercising on machines alone can be quite boring. Because of this fact, LA Fitness has integrated different kinds of sports in their fitness program for you to enjoy and play with your family and friends. They also have different cardio and weight machines for people who prefer this kind of exercise.

Another great thing about LA Fitness is that everybody is welcome to be a member. Whether you are a beginner or advanced in terms of fitness level, you can be sure that someone in LA Fitness will be able to help you with your workouts and the staff will also give you an exercise plan that is suitable for your fitness level.

With LA Fitness, you can be sure that you will be able to have fun while getting fit with their different fitness activities integrated in their fitness programs. The next time you get bored in a regular gym because of the regular routines, you should consider becoming a member of LA Fitness and experience getting fit while having fun.

THE FITNESS WORLD OF FITNESS PLANET

There's Gold Gym, Peak Fitness, and a string of other fitness centers and health clubs that are opening up their doors for everyone. And then, there's Planet Fitness. Planet fitness is a chain of fitness centers in the United States. Known for its 'Judgment Free Zone', it caters to the common person or the fitness neophytes who may feel conscious about their fitness needs and requirements.

The fitness club offers choices on exercise equipment and personal trainers who can assist members in their work-outs. There are a wide variety of machines aimed to build cardiovascular ability. Planet fitness centers offer a generally low price to its members. Those interested can take advantage of a $15 membership fee every month. Other perks of this fitness club is a Black Card membership that allows the member to use the facilities for free. There's also a guest allowance per day, a 50% discount on cool drinks and unlimited tanning for those enrolled in their home clubs.

There's a Planet Fitness Co-ed Zone and more private club for the women, the Women Zone. These innovations in programs offer a work-out package which includes a complete fitness assessment upon enrollment. In the assessment, the individual's fitness needs and requirements are analyzed, and they are given an exercise recommendation based on the results of the analysis. There are also 'acceleration' programs to speed up the individual's work-out plan, based on the results of their initial work-out programs. And as maintenance is important, the club also offers private personal training sessions where members can benefit the services of personal physical fitness trainers.

On the other hand, the club underscores a number of exercise rules and etiquettes that need to be observed among members and users. The club prohibits compound barbell exercises like deadlifts and bent over row exercises. Dumbbell use is restricted to a maximum of 80 pounds. The use of magnesium carbonate in heavy lifts is also prohibited. Exercise etiquette is strictly observed, which means no grunting, swearing or loud psyching up rituals. Excessive noise from bar drops is also prohibited. Members are warned of such violations by an alarm that rings every time a member breaks any of the rules.

And while some may see these rules as restrictive and ironic for a 'Judgment Free Zone', many are still willing to go for the club's reasonably-priced program, wide choice of exercise equipment and the other amenities the club offers.

The choice of enrolling yourself in a health and fitness club or gym like Planet Fitness is really yours to make. Serious fitness buffs would like to benefit of the amenities, the equipment, and the professional guidance that a gym like Planet Fitness offers. Of course, Planet Fitness tailors its services to the more sensitive, first-timers. But just like any other fitness and health club, Planet Fitness aims to serve you first, your body and your health!

Start Your Exercise Routine Slowly

Have you ever felt tired and stressed out from work and by the time you get home you see your three children running towards you asking you to play basketball with them? You refused and promised them that you will after you take a rest.

Instead of disappointing your children say "yes"! You will be surprised by the amount of energy you will have after that 30-minute activity.

Did you know that by exercising at a moderate pace for only 30 minutes, you would feel a lot better? It has been proven that this improves the appetite and sharpens your style in problem solving. You will also feel that it is easier to sleep at night if you do moderate exercises even for only 30 minutes every day.

Exercise helps in lifting your spirits and getting you out of any depression. It promotes self- discipline and has a positive impact how you perceive life. For first timers, it can be done for 15 minutes for 2 to 3 days a week. You can increase the time you spend once your body gets tuned up for it.

DON'T ever force your body! If you get hurt, stop. You can take a break from exercising for a few days and then you can start again but you need to start back at day 1.

Here are some moderate exercises you can do and enjoy:

1. Go Walking. Make use of your surroundings.

You can walk your dog, with your partner or child. Encourage your family to do walking exercises daily and you will find yourself burning calories while enjoying the surroundings and getting enough sunlight which is also good for you.

2. Discover the wonders of Yoga.

Yoga is one effective exercise that energizes not only your body but also your soul. You may want to learn even the basic yoga positions that are not too complicated but proven effective. A five-minute yoga exercise can perk you up and recharge your body with the energy you lost for the whole day. You relax and at the same time you stretch!

3. Engage yourself in sports.

Play basketball, football, baseball, tennis or badminton. Many doctors have recommended sports as an effective way to stay fit and healthy. Sports can also be done in moderation. Do not take it seriously. Shooting basketball with a friend is one moderate exercise that is also considered a sport.

4. Join exercise programs at work.

If you still do not have exercises programs at work, then why not start one? You can talk to your boss about it and start with your colleagues. You do not only lose calories but it is also one good way to bond with them. This can be done 30 minutes, 3 times a week.

5. Exercise while doing household chores.

Gardening, raking leaves, lawn mowing, doing the laundry, vacuuming and car washing are effective moderate exercises at home. Make use of these chores to sweat and burn calories. Instead of using machines and gadgets to perform these chores, why not do it with your hands and lose some fats?

Making exercise a part of your daily routine will surprise you by how many calories lose. Doing these moderate exercises the same amount every day can burn up to 150 to 1,000 calories a day!

More and more people are now attuned to their fitness needs. Whether it's an indoor or outdoor exercise activity, they will always take the chance to stay physically fit and healthy. Outdoor exercises are also popular nowadays. Like indoor exercises, you can get a lot of benefits like:

1. Little equipment is needed in order to have a good workout; but there are also exercises that don't require any equipment at all

2. No more obnoxious people or crowded gyms

3. No need to drive back and forth a fitness facility

4. You can enjoy the fresh air

5. Doesn't require special workout outfit or make-up

6. You get a lot of sunshine and vitamin D

7. You can work out anytime and anywhere

Some of the reasons for preferring outdoor exercises as a fitness routine may not be included on the list but whatever your reason, there are still other things to think about. Now that you know the benefits, the next step is to learn the different activities fit for the outdoors. There are seven top outdoor exercises; if you want to get all sweaty, feeling great and worn out, you can check out these exercises.

Lunges – this kind of exercise should be done in perfect form so that all your leg muscles, as well as your buttock muscles will work with every motion. You can also include some variations like standing lunges, alternative, elevated, walking, and rear lunges.

Pushups – this is truly an effective exercise for your upper body but very few people do this now because they prefer press machines. The push up is a productive exercise that doesn't require any equipment. The basic movements include standard, wide, and close grips. By doing the three basic movements alternately, you can stimulate the muscles on your shoulders, chest, and triceps. You can achieve easier movement by elevating your hands; for harder movement, try elevating your feet. If you're brave enough, you can try clapping and bounce pushups.

Squats – doing squats the proper way can provide incredible power. Its effectiveness has been lost due to inappropriate form, improper instruction, and laziness. You can do variations like one leg, standing, pile, wide-stance, and overhead squat. By doing repetitions, you can feel your legs getting tired which means its taking its effect.

Step ups – if you do this exercise properly, then you're doing a brutal exercise. A bench will do as your equipment, and all you have to do is to step up and down. Just make sure that your head is up at all times and your back is in a straight position. This is also a great cardio exercise.

Chin ups – also called pull ups; use a tree branch or any playground equipment that allows you to pull yourself up and down. You can repeat this exercise as many times as you like.

Uphill sprints – try this exercise only if you can do a 100 meter dash. This is carried out by running uphill. Find a decent-sized hill and run up fast. Then walk right down. Just keep on repeating.

Duck walks – walk like a duck; squat down and stay put, then start walking. Repeat as necessary.

Doing outdoor exercises the right way is hard, but the benefits you can get can't be easily ignored.

Hardcore Training

Many people think about building muscles as abandoning life outside the gym and devoting hours in the gym like a monk in a monastery. Perhaps the only way to chisel the body into a hot muscular physique is by toiling hour by hour over the rusty iron day in, day out and year in, year out.

Although hard work is truly required, extreme fitness demands one to be a slave of the iron weights. Full-body work outs can make you progress and fit easily into your schedule. This is very convenient if you are looking to achieve extreme fitness but find it hard to hold on to a single workout routine.

Genuine full-body work outs make for a maximum muscle contraction using heavy weights. Make room for full recovery so you can actually grow and continue to train hard plus it also prevents burnout which is inevitable due to excess training.

So if you are ready for extreme fitness, here is all there is to know about full body work out:

A full-body work out is a time saver. The biggest plus about having the whole body trained at once is less frequently at the gym; perhaps around two to three times for every seven days would be enough.

Another advantage of working out the entire body all at once is that you need not spend two or more hours of strenuous exercise in the gym for every session; one only spends one hour in the gym for every session. So that's just three to four hours per week in the gym. With full-body work outs, it is all about the quality of exercise you do per session and not the quantity, nor even the amount of time you allot per session.

Full-body work outs boost the cardiovascular system for extreme fitness. You must allot two to four sets for every body part into the one hour session. Jam packed with exercising, each one hour session then gets the heart and the rest of the cardiovascular system pumping and up to speed in a flash.

Now feeling pumped up, next find out what rules do you have to follow when engaging in a full- body work out:

Training commences only once every two to three days. What is great about this is that there is time spared during rest days so that one can indulge in a few cardio exercise sessions instead of depending on cardio exercises one normally does at the end of each work out session which after all, are not at all very effective.

Heavy lifting is strongly advised; contrary to popular belief, especially among athletes. It is not good to get trapped on training to conserve energy for later in the routine. What is true is that you cannot achieve optimal progress if you do not train heavy, no matter which program.

One exercise only per muscle group. This is very easy to follow and is also important. Doing basic exercises which are also intense means you do not have to do another different exercise for that body part.

Keep your work out short. Resistance training affects the natural hormones of the body connected to muscle building. Intense exercising boosts the testosterone levels and long work outs increase those of catabolic cortical. Sixty minutes of work out allows you to get the best of both worlds.

Now with this convenient and powerful workout regimen, one can now truly experience extreme fitness.

Get The Most of Your Workout

1. Stop and Go

If you play a sport that requires a full sprint, remember that a full sprint strains the muscles of the lower body. To combat this, do stop-and-go exercises. For example, run 30 meters at about 80 percent of your effort, slow to a jog for 5 to 10 meters, then run again for another 30 meters.

Repeat this process five times.

2. On bended knees

Almost 3 out of 4 ACL injuries occur when players are landing or turning. If your knees are bent instead of straight, the risk of injury is greatly reduced according to a report in the JAAOS (Journal of the American Academy of Orthopedic Surgeons).

3. Cool down

Heatstroke is not something that can be easily cured like headaches. To avoid it, stay cool and hydrated. Be sure the combined temp and humidity is less than 160. This is according to Dr. Dave Janda of the IPSM.

4. Get the proper equipment

Badly fitting gears or ill sized equipment can be a cause of training injuries. The extra money spent on proper equipment goes a long way.

5. Do it the right way

Bad technique is just as bad as, bad equipment. Seek advice from pros and trainer, their advice is invaluable to your exercises or training.

6. Go West (or whichever direction)

If you're playing or training in multiple directions, your warm up should also. Move sideways, backward, forward and all the motions you might be doing. This allows your body to be prepared.

7. Have yourself filmed

The camera doesn't lie. Show your video to a person well verse in your training, so he can give a critic of your fitness regimen.

8. Loosen the shoulders

Even a slightly injured rotator cuff can shut down the function of a shoulder. You might want to include stretching to protect your rotator cuffs.

9. Take an early dip

Schedule your swimming sessions early as there are less people in the pool, and the less of everything in the pool.

10. Protect yourself

Wearing custom-fit mouth guards reduces the risk of injuries by as much as 82 percent, according to a study at UNC at Chapel Hill. Plunk out the cash for a custom-fit mouth guard and it'll last for years including your smile and teeth.

11. Smooth out your tendon

Inquire about ultrasound needle therapy. This procedure is minimally by using ultrasound to guide a needle. The needle smooth's the bone, breaks up calcifications, and fixes scar tissue. 13 out of 20 patients saw improvement, and the session takes only about 15 minutes of your time.

12. Buy your running shoes after work.

Shop in the evening, the feet are swollen after a day of work. It approximates how your feet will be after three miles of running.

13. Do off road running.

If the surface is unstable, it trains the ankles to be stable.

14. Know where you're going.

Whether its biking, or skiing, be sure to have a dry run down any path first. A lot of injuries can be avoided when you're familiar with the route.

15. Train hard.

Anxiety reduces your peripheral vision by three degrees and slows the reaction time by almost 120 milliseconds, according to an article of the Journal of Sports Sciences. When the going gets difficult, the veteran athlete relies on skills they've trained for and practiced. It keeps them cooler under pressure, widening their vision so they can see react much faster.

Pick Your Fitness Routine

Many people today are now getting more and more concerned about their health. With the alarming increase in heart related diseases and diabetes and the United States having been nicknamed as the fattest country in the world, you have every right to be concerned about your body. You have to consider that your body plays a major role on how you live your daily life.

By having a healthy body, you will be able to enjoy life more. You also need to consider that having diabetes and heart related disease will also affect your family's life. So, if you want a healthy body, you have to turn off your TV, get off your comfortable recliner and start exercising. You also need to consider that you have to have a proper diet In order to maintain your body's health and prevent it from acquiring different kinds of diseases.

Today, there are thousands of gyms located all over the United States. You can consider enrolling in one of these gyms in order to get a perfectly healthy body. You have to consider that by exercising, you will not only have a healthy body and a healthy heart, but you will also have a great looking body that you can proudly show off.

All you need to do is find the right fitness program for you. Gyms today have professional fitness experts or fitness trainers that can give you the right fitness program for you. If you just want to maintain a healthy heart and have a well-toned body, the right fitness program for you will concentrate more on cardiovascular exercises plus a diet program that will help you maintain your heart's health.

If you want to have stronger muscles, you have to consider that weight training plus intensive cardiovascular exercises are required in your fitness program. You also need to consider that there are different fitness programs for different kinds of people. Even children have their very own fitness programs and even the elderly have their very own fitness program.

You need to consider that you fitness program will depend on the current state your body is in. If you are too fat or overweight, you will first enter a weight loss fitness program. After you finish your weight loss fitness program and have reached the required weight, you will now enter a different and more advanced fitness program that will concentrate on strength and endurance training. However, if you are too thin, you will enter a weight gain fitness program.

As you can see, there are different kinds of fitness programs available today. You have to consider that the right fitness program for you will depend entirely on your current health status and your body status. These are some of the things you have to consider when choosing a fitness program for you.

Chapter 7- Reap the Benefits of Hard Training

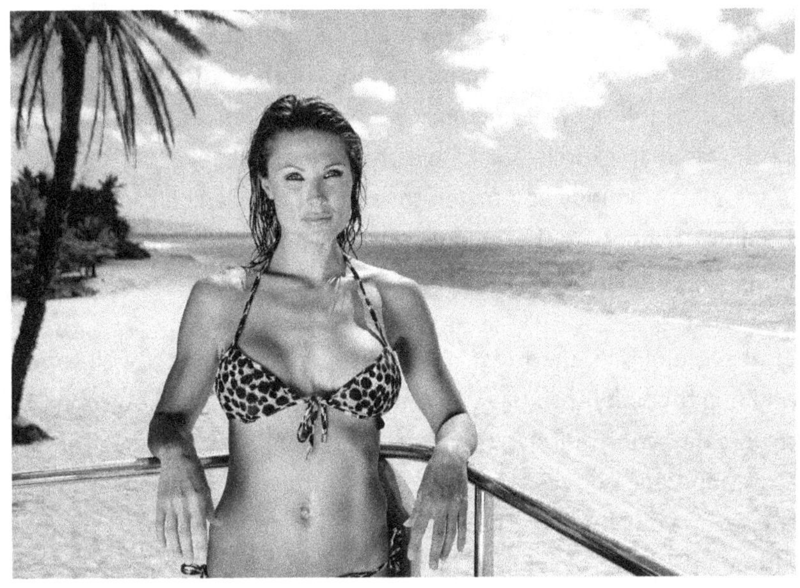

In today's society, many people are now getting more and more concerned about their physical appearance. Besides, having a good looking body means that you can attract more of the opposite sex. This is why many people go through liposuction surgery or experiment with their body by trying out different kinds of diets. Although liposuction surgery can give you a thinner and better looking body, you have to consider that this process won't necessarily develop your body. The process will involve sucking out fats from a specific part of your body and the surgeon will "sculpt" your body to get a better looking figure.

In dieting, you should consider that this can be very dangerous for your body as it can deprive the body of the nutrients it needs. Some diets say that you shouldn't eat carbohydrates, which your body needs in order to have energy. Some diets suggest fasting which also means depriving your body of the essential nutrients it needs. With the proper diet plus fitness training, you will be able to obtain a well-toned body with all the health benefits because fitness training actually keeps your heart pumping, therefore, making it healthy.

There are quite a lot of fitness training methods available today. You have to choose the fitness training method that will suit your needs. If you like body building, you have to concentrate more on cardiovascular exercises and weight lifting. However, if you only want a healthy body and a well-toned one, you can consider fitness training exercises that concentrate more on cardiovascular exercises and a little on weight training.

Fitness training is the most natural way of obtaining a well-toned and healthy body. You have to remember that muscles burn fat. By developing your muscles it will burn fat at the same time. The fat stored in your body is what keeps your muscles working. Think of the fat in your body as the fuel for your muscles. This is why that although dieting alone can give you a slimmer body, it will lack strength because you are depriving your muscles of fat.

You have to consider that the human body needs fat in order for it to work properly. However, you have to use those fats in order for you to not have that "extra padding" or those "love handles".

You can try hunting for your own food in the wilderness as what the humans before did that is both an exercise and a necessity. Technology has contributed to obesity and being overweight. The best way that you can use your fat and at the same time develop your body's muscles is through fitness training.

Make Training Feel Like Play

When you ask someone to workout with you, you will usually hear the word "no". Besides, working out is boring. Maybe even you will consider that working out is boring and rather do fun things than spending time at the gym doing some boring workout routines. You have to consider that more and more people are putting up with the boring workout routines because of the alarming increase of heart related diseases and obesity. You have to consider that you have to take care of your body in order to live a happier and more satisfying life.

You and only you are responsible for maintaining your body's health. This is why you have to do fitness workouts in order to keep your body in top working condition. Failing to do so will result in a disease-ridden life where you and your family will suffer. So, while you are still not experiencing diseases because of being overweight, such as diabetes and heart diseases, you have to start doing fitness workout in order to keep your body healthy plus giving you the benefit of having a great looking body that you can show off during summers at the beach.

If you find regular fitness workout routines very boring, there are quite a lot of fitness workouts that you can do to make working out more fun. There are fun activities that you can do where you can definitely enjoy and at the same time, get a great quality fitness workout experience.

Most people consider that fitness workouts are only limited at the gym. However, you have to consider thinking out of the box and start being creative. Active sports such as swimming, golf, tennis, football, and basketball is a fun sport that can give you great quality fitness workout experience. For example, if you like to play tennis, there are quite a lot of tennis schools available that can teach you how to play. You can even include your family in this fun activity and all of you can have fun while at the same time, promote fitness.

If you are not sports minded or you can't think of any sport that can be fun for you, you can also consider dancing as a great fitness workout experience. You can try and enroll in dance classes. Although some people think that dancing is easy, you have to consider that it's not. Dancing is quite difficult and can be very stressful for your body as it will require you to run, walk, and jump around in the dance floor to do those dance moves. Dancing can definitely be a great fitness workout alternative if you find regular gym workouts boring. Dancing is also fun especially if both you and your significant other enroll in the same classes.

These are just some of the examples that can make fitness workout more fun and more enjoyable. There are still quite a lot of activities out there that you can do for fun and at the same time, give you a great quality workout. There are belly dancing activities, there are hiking and camping activities, there are rock climbing activities and a lot more. All you need to do is find one that interests you and be creative.

10 Tips on Stretching

Before fitness training, it is important to warm-up and does stretching exercises to prevent accidents and enhance the output during the training. There are also a number of precautionary measures and tips to serve as guidelines when doing fitness exercises. Here are some of them.

1. To increase your flexibility and to avoid injuries, stretch before and after workout. Almost everyone knows that stretching before a workout prevents injuries during the exercises, but only few people

know that stretching after workout, when muscles are still warm, can increase flexibility.

2. Hold your stretching position for more than 60 seconds to increase flexibility. While holding your position for 20 seconds is enough for warm ups, holding each position for at least 60 seconds will develop the body's flexibility.

3. Do not go into a stretching position then immediately return to the relaxed position, and do it repeatedly. This is more appropriately termed as bouncing while in a position. When stretching, hold that position for several seconds, and then slowly relax. You may do this exercise repeatedly this way. Bouncing or forcing yourself into a position during stretching can strain or damage some joints or muscles.

4. Work slowly in increments instead of immediately prior to doing the hardest exercise or position.

5. Make sure that you have stretched or warmed up all muscle groups. For some people, even if they have strong bodies, they tend to neglect the neck when stretching. Stretching the neck muscles can be as simple as placing the palm of one's hand against the front of the head and pushing it. Then, do the same to the sides and the back of the head.

6. Stretch regularly to continually increase your range of movements and your level of flexibility and strength.

7. Workout considering only your capabilities and not of others. Do not force yourself to do exercises that you are not yet capable of just because there are people who can do it. Increase your limits slowly. Listen to your body. There are days when your body may be

too tired that you may have to consider reducing your range of motion.

8. Learn to rest. Rest in between sets and stations to make sure that the body has enough time to recover its energy. Also, it is advisable that you don't work the same muscle groups consecutively for two days. The muscles grow during the period when you rest and not when you are working out.

9. Do aerobic exercises to strengthen your heart. Aerobic exercises are those activities that use much oxygen for fuel. This includes cardiovascular exercises such as skipping rope, running or swimming.

10. Music may help you when you want to train for longer periods or to increase your intensity. You can use mp3 players, CD players or lightweight am radio receivers for this. Just make sure that you brought your headset with you so you wouldn't disturb people who don't prefer music while exercising.

Apart from preventing injuries and increasing one's limit, it is also said that stretching is good for a tired body and also for a stressed mind and spirit.

Make Fitness a Priority

The human body is considered fit if it's mental and physical health are good, it strictly follows proper habits, diets, and exercises, and can handle and deal with everyday stresses.

You should nurture your body with proper nutrition to function well and stay healthy. Important minerals, vitamins, and foods must be provided to achieve overall fitness. Keep in mind that good spiritual, mental, and physical health is the real meaning of fitness.

Body fitness occurs if all the processes of the body associated with mental and physical state are functioning at its peak levels. However, this is not only a one day task. It does not necessarily mean going to a gym or simply taking a walk in a park.

There are several factors that must be considered when talking about body fitness. Daily necessities as well as body conditioning are needed.

Physical exercise absolutely helps the body in becoming strong. All parts of your body need to function as a whole. Therefore, the absence of one factor can fail your entire fitness needs. Take for instance; you only focus on maintaining your weight and meeting cardiovascular needs. You forgot that your body is not only composed of your heart. All your other organs should also be functioning well. Body fitness is not only achieving a beautiful figure but replenishing what was depleted from the body due to daily activities. Physical exercises should benefit your entire body.

Available resources must be used wisely. Educating yourself about bodily needs for maintaining a fit body is also important. If you have an unhealthy body, you need to dig deeply for its causes. In fact, becoming fit again is not easy as you could observe that what makes your body unfit is several years of body abuse from bad habits, poor nutrition, and lack of physical exercises.

You should also know the difference between wellness and fitness since some have misconception about it. Being well and being fit is entirely different and have exclusive conditions, but both are essential in maintaining vitality and health. A fitness counselor or licensed fitness instructor at a fitness club or local gym can test your fitness levels, while wellness is determined by optimum functioning of your immune systems.

Beyond the Diet with Healthy Diet Recipes

The body maintains its balance if both fitness and wellness are in its maximum levels. Generally, nutritional intake affects the ability of the mind, body, and staying well. If this is combined with healthy eating, clean living, and regular exercise, then it will result to total wellness and fitness.

Giving proper attention on the physical needs of every body parts can also result to total body fitness. Never forget that these parts are working in unison with one another. In order for the limbs to function at its peak levels, two hands, two eyes, two feet, and other parts are important.

Your physical body works better compared to any invented machine. It's more powerful and complex, thus it can take more abuse yet continuously operate without meeting its everyday requirements for a few days. If you put body fitness first in your life, then your body can do its work tremendously well.

Fit and Single

It is a fact that being single and free is a lot of fun. However, you have to realize that you still need to socialize in order for you to meet new people and make new friends or perhaps even meet that special someone you have always been looking for.

Dating and socializing isn't the only thing you should worry about. You also need to consider that you have to maintain a healthy and great looking body in order to enjoy life to the fullest. Today, there are fitness programs available exclusively for singles. You can enjoy life through meeting other singles and making new friends and at the same time, workout for a healthier and better looking body.

There are exercise programs especially made for singles today. By joining these programs, you will be able to have more fun exercising than before. This is because these kinds of programs are integrated with fun activities that you can do with other singles. There are cross country mountain biking, swimming activities and other sports activities.

As you can see, it can be a lot of fun exercising. You have to consider that companies that offer these kinds of activities aren't dating companies. These companies offer fitness activities for singles in order for singles to enjoy working out more. You have to consider that hiking or biking alone can be quite boring. So, what these companies do is that they organize a group of singles to meet and do fitness activities they enjoy together.

First of all, you have to join a company that offers fitness single programs. You have to state your preferences, you sexual orientation, your age, and also state the fitness activity, such as hiking, mountain biking, or any activity that you enjoy doing most. It is the company's responsibility to pair you with a group of singles that also shares your interest in the fitness activity and also pair you within your age group.

Joining fitness single programs can be quite an enjoyable experience. Besides, by joining fitness single programs, you will never have to do your favorite fitness activity alone again. As you can see, it can be quite fun to join these activities. If you enjoy boxing, you will be paired to another single that enjoys boxing too. You can spar and enjoy your favorite activity while socializing and getting a healthier and better looking body. Who knows, maybe in these activities you will meet the man or woman of your dreams. You have to consider that you will already share a common interest to the person you are paired with because you will already do the same activities that they also enjoy. All you need to do is develop the relationship further.

These are some of the things you have to know about the fitness single programs available today. Here, you will have the chance to make new friends or even better, meet the person of your dreams and enjoy doing your activities with him or her forever.

Targeting Your Fitness Goals

Being fit always brings to mind the idea of bulging muscles, superman strength and a to-die-for athletic built. Fitness more importantly means the body's resistance level and stamina for physical activities. Peak fitness means achieving the fullest and the optimum potential of your strength and stamina in your activities.

Contrary to what most people think that peak fitness is only for the young, any middle-aged individual can still achieve peak fitness given the conditions of his body. Achieving peak fitness does not only mean working on a good body built and having the energy and the muscles to do hard, manual, physical labor. It also means following good health habits designed not only to build and develop your muscles, but to sustain your body with the energy and the requirements needed to performance your tasks to your fullest potential.

Maintain a balanced quantity of calories in your body. Don't stop eating calorie-rich food just because you're trying to cut back on your calories and lose weight. Calories are used in the performance of simple, ordinary tasks. Load up on fiber. It is important for good digestion and bowel movement. Fiber-rich food like wheat bread, unpolished rice, vegetables and fruits give you a feeling of fullness, which reduces the tendency to overeat. Of course, don't forget your greens. Maintaining a daily vegetable and fruit intake provides you with the necessary vitamins and minerals to beef up your stamina and resistance to disease, ultimately leading to your body's peak fitness.

Avoid a sedentary lifestyle. Be mobile. Exercise and be active. Keeping your body used to physical activity and an active lifestyle develops the muscles and strengthens your body's capacity to do certain tasks. Sedate individuals do not only gain more flab in their middle; they are also more prone to injuries and illness. Ten minutes of routine exercise everyday – from something as simple as taking the stairs to stretching and working on the treadmill can help your body maintain its peak fitness level. Of course, remember not to abuse your body. Have moments for lazing around and relaxing those muscles of yours. Too much and too little of anything is bad.

Give yourself enough sleep. Sleep is important as it allows your body to rejuvenate, the tissues to heal, the brain and other organs to slow down in their function. A good night's sleep spells more energy the next day, a more enthusiastic, active you. Enough sleep allows you and your body to function optimally, to your fullest potential. It is the body's means to recharge itself.

The easiest measure to check your peak fitness level is your body's ability to respond to stress. More so, peak fitness is your body's ability to respond to emergencies. A well-oiled machine should be able to function without the 'clicks' and the 'thuds'. Our body should be able to do its work in much the same way.

Do You Need a Personal Trainer?

These days, not only movie stars could afford them. No, we're not talking of designer clothes and shoes. We're talking about personal fitness trainers that only movie stars and millionaires could afford in the past. These days, anyone who's a member of a gym can have a personal fitness trainer who creates a routine workout just for them.

Most people who are serious about their fitness plans would insist on the services of a trainer on the grounds that a personal trainer provides the proper guidance and advices the individual of the needs in their exercises. They can prepare a set of exercises that you can do in the gym and even at home. With a trainer, the individual is more focused on his work-out goals. There is someone who will encourage him/her and help point out the parts of the body that needs work-out and toning.

Sessions may range from a hundred to a thousand dollars, depending on the extent of services to be provided by your trainer. While others may charge a certain fee for a set number of work-outs, others charge for individual sessions. But the market for personal fitness trainers has significantly expanded with the increasing number of fitness buffs and health enthusiasts. As a fitness trainer, your market would be professionals, athletes and people who want to get fit and stay in shape.

There's also a potential market for people undergoing therapy, those with high blood pressure and diabetics who needs to have a physically fit body to maintain their health. There are also those who need a trainer or coach for specialized sports related skills like aerobics and karate.

Those thinking of a career as a physical fitness trainer should be equipped with the basics of anatomy, physiology, nutrition, metabolism, design and implementation of fitness plans, health safety and first aid – topics which are taught at fitness training schools. These training schools may also provide specializations in different types of physical activities like yoga, strength training, running etc. There are also lessons on designing programs for people with special health needs and issues – the diabetics, heart disease patients and patients with back injuries.

Trainers can earn as low as $16,000 to as much as $80,000, depending on their experience and skills. Of course, personal trainers to prominent personalities like athletes and movie stars earn more.

If you're thinking of making this a career, remember that a physical fitness trainer provides more than just exercise and work-out plans. A physical fitness trainer is sensitive to the needs and conditions of his client. They are good motivators who can effectively encourage and promote healthy living and fitness to their clients. The reason why most solitary fitness buffs fail in their work-outs is because of the lack of motivation from a companion. The fitness trainer fills in this role of motivator – one who will keep them going even when they think the work-out's not working.

With a career as a physical fitness trainer, you get more than just a healthy and fit body. You may get to rub elbows with the stars too!

The Right Trainer Has a Lot to Teach

One of the biggest obstacles to staying on track for fitness is losing motivation. People just starting an exercise program can find themselves quickly tired of the same routine. Keeping exercise appealing and maintaining a good fitness perspective is the key to long-term success.

If you have to watch the exact same episode of your favorite television show every day for the rest of your life, you would probably be banging your head against the wall by the end of the week. You would change the channel, pick up a book, or do anything you could to avoid something you once enjoyed.

Yet, many people starting a fitness program feel compelled to follow the same routine, day after day after day, and consequently fall off the exercise wagon due to sheer boredom. That is why most people want the services of a fitness trainer in order to provide them the different portions of the fitness program in a livelier style.

Fitness trainers are experts in analyzing and creating a fitness program that is right for you. They are the ones who will calculate your appropriateness to a certain program with regards to your "fitness level," create the program according to your specific needs, and keep you stimulated and inspired by giving you activities that will not bore you. But then again, as with other entities included in the fitness world, not all fitness trainers are created equal. They may vary from the different trainings that they have, the health education they have acquired, and the skills that they have learned. Hence, it is important to consider some factors that will determine if a certain fitness trainer is right for you.

Here is how:

1. Certification

Like any item or product, the quality is sometimes measured and determined through the certification that goes with it. Hence, before you choose your fitness trainer, it is important to verify if the trainer is duly certified by a highly regarded fitness association. It is also best to choose a trainer that has a CPR certification or first aid qualifications.

2. Education/Trainings

Be sure to choose a fitness trainer who had acquired an adequate training and education as far as health and physical fitness is concerned. Even though it is not necessary, trainers who have acquired education connected with health or any other related field will definitely have an edge over the others.

3. Knows how to give the right attention

A good fitness trainer should know how to provide his or her client an undivided attention whenever their session is going on. In this way, the trainer will be able to focus more on the details that needs attention and immediate considerations.

4. Knows how to track development

It is best to choose a fitness trainer that knows how to track his or her client's progress as far as fitness is concerned. In this way, the trainer will be able to generate new activities and trainings designated for a particular result of the client.

5. Good Personality

Since you will be dealing most with your fitness trainer, it is best if you will look for somebody with a pleasing personality, somebody whom you can be comfortable. It is best to hire the services of somebody whom you can easily get along with.

The services of a fitness center and the contributions it can give you while working out on those belly fats are, indeed, one of the best help that you can get from a professional person who knows what he is doing. Hence, it is best to choose the best person who can give you the best services that you need so that you will never get bored again.

ABOUT THE AUTHOR

Christopher Miller encountered health issues as a baby. He had immune system deficiency. His parents was really worried then. By time Christopher was a teenager, his parents decided that he needs to get active like engaging in sports perhaps. Christopher joined the local football team and since then, he really made sure to keep his body sound and healthy.

Christopher is now a sought after fitness instructor in the country. Christopher is married and they have 3 healthy boys.

www.ingramcontent.com/pod-product-compliance
Lightning Source LLC
Chambersburg PA
CBHW070033260726
48658CB00002B/612